PARKINSON'S DISEASE DIET COOKBOOK: FOR SENIORS AND BEGINNERS

Enjoy Relief from Symptoms, Improved Brain Health, Stabilized Blood Levels, Reduced Inflammation in the Body, and Boosted Energy Levels

Steve Bryant, MD, RD

Copyright Page

Table of Contents

Introduction

Parkinson's disease, alternatively known as Morbus Parkinson, shaking palsy, or Parkinson's, is a progressive neurological disorder that predominantly affects the elderly demographic, although it can manifest at any age. This condition is characterized by a wide array of symptoms, with motor impairments such as tremors, bradykinesia (slowed movement), rigidity, and postural instability being the most prominent. Additionally, non-motor symptoms like cognitive impairment, mood disturbances, sleep disturbances, and autonomic dysfunction often accompany the motor symptoms, further complicating the management of the disease.

The precise cause of Parkinson's disease remains elusive, despite extensive scientific investigation into its pathogenesis. While genetic predisposition and environmental factors are believed to play significant roles, the exact interplay between these factors and the mechanisms underlying neuronal degeneration in the brain remains incompletely understood. Researchers continue to explore various hypotheses, including the involvement of oxidative stress, mitochondrial dysfunction, inflammation, and protein aggregation, particularly the accumulation of misfolded alpha-synuclein protein in the form of Lewy bodies, which are characteristic pathological features of Parkinson's disease.

Moreover, Parkinson's disease is not solely a motor disorder; it impacts multiple aspects of an individual's life, including cognition, emotional well-being, and overall quality of life. As the disease progresses, individuals may experience increasing difficulty in performing activities of daily living independently, leading to a significant burden on both patients and their caregivers.

Despite the challenges posed by Parkinson's disease, ongoing research efforts aim to develop more effective treatments to alleviate symptoms, slow disease progression, and ultimately find a cure. Additionally, multidisciplinary approaches, including pharmacological interventions, physical therapy, occupational therapy, speech therapy, and psychosocial support, are essential in managing the multifaceted nature of this complex condition and improving the overall quality of life for individuals living with Parkinson's disease.

Chapter 1: What exactly constitutes Parkinson's disease?

Parkinson's disease, also known as Morbus Parkinson or shaking palsy, stands as a complex neurological disorder that predominantly affects the aging demographic, posing significant challenges to mobility and daily functioning. Despite decades of scientific inquiry, the precise etiology of this condition remains elusive, with multiple factors likely contributing to its onset and progression.

This debilitating illness, once diagnosed, often heralds a life-altering journey for individuals and their families. While the disease itself is currently considered incurable, advancements in medical research and therapeutic interventions have significantly improved the quality of life for many patients. Although the pathophysiological mechanisms driving Parkinson's disease remain enigmatic, the gradual and insidious nature of its progression underscores the importance of early detection and intervention strategies.

In the face of this formidable neurological challenge, individuals grappling with Parkinson's disease often find themselves navigating a myriad of physical, cognitive, and emotional hurdles. Yet, despite the pervasive impact of the illness on daily life, many individuals with Parkinson's disease continue to exhibit remarkable resilience and tenacity, striving to maintain a sense of independence and purpose.

Indeed, the management of Parkinson's disease extends far beyond the realm of pharmacotherapy. While medications play a pivotal role in mitigating symptoms and slowing disease progression, a multidisciplinary approach encompassing physical therapy, occupational therapy, speech therapy, and psychosocial support is essential for optimizing patient outcomes and enhancing overall well-being.

Furthermore, the journey of living with Parkinson's disease is fraught with uncertainties and challenges, both for the individual affected and their caregivers. From navigating the complexities of medication management and adjusting to fluctuations in symptom severity to grappling with issues of stigma and social isolation, the journey of Parkinson's disease encompasses a broad spectrum of experiences and emotions.

However, amidst the trials and tribulations, there exists a profound sense of resilience and camaraderie within the Parkinson's community. Through advocacy efforts, support groups, and ongoing research endeavors, individuals affected by Parkinson's disease continue to inspire hope and drive positive change.

In conclusion, Parkinson's disease stands as a multifaceted neurological condition that profoundly impacts the lives of those affected. While the journey may be fraught with challenges, it is also characterized by resilience, strength, and a shared sense of purpose in striving for improved

treatments and ultimately, a cure.

What are the typical motor manifestations of Parkinson's disease?

The motor symptoms associated with Parkinson's disease revolve around alterations in an individual's movement patterns. Those grappling with the disorder often encounter stiffness and tremors. As Parkinson's advances, mobility and speech may become challenging. Here, we delve into some of the prevalent motor symptoms of Parkinson's disease:

Tremor:

The initial symptom that usually catches attention is tremor, as described by Dr. Lynda Nwabuobi, MD, an assistant professor of clinical neurology at Weill Cornell Parkinson's Disease and Movement

Disorders Institute. This trembling typically manifests at rest, where the affected limb appears relaxed but exhibits shaking. Initially, tremors might localize to one side of the body, commonly in the hand, foot, or leg. It's also plausible to experience tremors in the jaw, chin, mouth, or tongue. Progression of the disease might lead to tremors in the opposite side of the body as well. While tremor signifies a symptom of Parkinson's disease, it could stem from other disorders like multiple sclerosis, stress, exertion, or specific medications. Hence, consulting a physician upon noticing tremors or any other potential symptoms of Parkinson's disease is advisable.

Rigidity:

Another primary motor symptom of Parkinson's disease is rigidity, characterized by stiffness or tightness in the limbs. Initially, individuals might attribute their stiffness to an injury, arthritis, or aging. However, rigidity associated with Parkinson's tends to be more severe compared to typical stiffness from arthritis or aging. This stiffness may affect one or both sides of the body and can limit range of motion, leading to joint and muscle discomfort.

Bradykinesia:

Bradykinesia, indicating slowness of movement, significantly impacts mobility and initiation of actions such as standing from a chair. It may also alter facial expressions, resulting in what's known as facial masking. Signs of bradykinesia in

Parkinson's disease encompass difficulties with fine motor coordination, slower physical actions, reduced blink rate, shuffling while walking, and diminished arm swing during locomotion.

Posture Changes:

Poor posture and instability typically manifest as late-stage symptoms of Parkinson's disease. Individuals may struggle to maintain an upright, balanced posture and become more prone to falls. This symptom includes rounded shoulders, decreased curvature of the lower back, and forward-leaning of the body or head.

What are the symptoms of Parkinson's disease that do not involve motor functions?

While Parkinson's disease is commonly associated with changes in movement, a wide array of non-motor symptoms also exist. These encompass various alterations in a person's health and well-being that can stem from Parkinson's. These symptoms, sometimes overshadowing tremors, rigidity, and slow movement, deserve close attention when identifying the disorder in someone. Here's a comprehensive look at some of the non-motor symptoms associated with Parkinson's disease:

Difficulty speaking:

People with Parkinson's may undergo shifts in their vocalization and communication patterns. This alteration may partly result from bradykinesia and cognitive changes, making speech issues both motor and non-motor symptoms of the disease. Specifically, you might notice a softer, breathier voice with a monotone quality. As the disease progresses, speech may become more rapid, with words blending together to the point of sounding unintelligible. Slurring, mumbling, or trailing off are also indicative of Parkinson's disease. It's crucial to note that speech difficulties could also be a consequence of stroke or other conditions and not exclusively indicative of Parkinson's.

Loss of smell:

A diminished sense of smell or hyposmia can serve as an early sign of Parkinson's disease, sometimes preceding a formal diagnosis by years. The pathology of Parkinson's begins long before motor symptoms manifest, often up to 30 years prior, according to experts. Individuals with Parkinson's may report a long-standing lack of smell when discussing their medical history. However, since this symptom might not significantly impact daily life, it often goes unnoticed or is attributed to other causes like allergies.

Sleep disturbances:

Approximately 75% of Parkinson's patients experience sleep-related issues, including insomnia. Addressing sleep problems is crucial, as poor sleep can lead to decreased well-being. Acting out dreams is an early sleep-related symptom that can emerge years before diagnosis. Additionally, medications used to manage Parkinson's symptoms may disrupt sleep patterns, necessitating medication adjustments to enhance quality of life.

Anxiety and depression:

Changes in mental health are common non-motor symptoms of Parkinson's, with roughly half of patients experiencing depression at some point, and about 40% developing an anxiety disorder. These conditions can stem from the emotional strain of coping with a chronic illness or from neurotransmitter imbalances directly related to Parkinson's.

Psychosis:

Hallucinations and delusions affect over half of Parkinson's patients during the disease's course. While the exact cause is uncertain, these symptoms may result from medication side effects or changes in the brain over time.

Cognitive changes:

In older adults, cognitive decline is a common non-motor symptom of Parkinson's, characterized by difficulties in executive function. These may include challenges in planning and executing tasks, concentration, memory, decision-making, and word retrieval. Early onset of these symptoms, preceding motor symptoms, might suggest a different disorder such as Lewy body dementia.

Other non-motor symptoms:

Beyond the aforementioned, Parkinson's may manifest in various other non-motor symptoms like urinary incontinence, vision changes, weight fluctuations, apathy, fatigue, constipation, nausea, small handwriting, swallowing difficulties, breathing problems, dizziness, and vertigo. However, it's essential to remember that these symptoms aren't exclusive to Parkinson's and could indicate other health issues, underscoring the importance of consulting a physician for proper diagnosis and management.

Chapter 2: The origins of Parkinson's Disease

Despite considerable understanding of the symptoms associated with Parkinson's disease, a fundamental question persists: What are the underlying causes of Parkinson's disease?

Unfortunately, there's no straightforward answer to this question. "We don't have a single cause," explains Dr. Lynda Nwabuobi, an assistant professor of clinical neurology at Weill Cornell Parkinson's Disease and Movement Disorders Institute. "But based on our research and knowledge, we understand that Parkinson's disease results from a complex interplay between the aging brain, genetic factors, and environmental influences."

Here, with the insights provided by medical professionals, we delve deeper into some of the factors that may contribute to the development of Parkinson's disease or increase one's risk of developing this neurodegenerative disorder.

Age

While aging itself does not directly cause Parkinson's disease, being an older individual is the most significant risk factor for this neurological disorder, according to Dr. Nwabuobi. Why is this the case? One explanation is that as individuals age, their brain cells become more susceptible to damage, much like other cells in the body. Additionally, changes in gene expression over time can lead to alterations in cellular activity that ultimately contribute to the development of Parkinson's.

Typically, Parkinson's is diagnosed in individuals in their 60s, and the likelihood of diagnosis increases with age. However, there are instances of early-onset Parkinson's, occurring before the age of 50, which accounts for approximately 4% of diagnosed cases. In such cases, the disease is more likely to have a genetic basis.

Genetics

Genetic factors contribute to Parkinson's disease in approximately 10% to 15% of cases, as per the

Parkinson's Foundation. However, genetic research in this field is still in its infancy, and experts have yet to fully understand the role genes play in the development of the disease. "While many gene mutations have been identified, we are just scratching the surface," notes Dr. Nwabuobi.

The first connection between genetics and Parkinson's was established in 1997 by researchers at the National Institutes of Health, who found that mutations in the SNCA gene (PARK 1), responsible for encoding the protein alpha-synuclein, were linked to the disease. Specifically, they discovered that alpha-synuclein aggregates into clumps called Lewy bodies within the brain cells of individuals with Parkinson's. Another mutation associated with Parkinson's occurs in the LRRK2 gene, with at least 20 known mutations identified. Individuals of Ashkenazi Jewish and North African Berber descent are particularly susceptible to this gene mutation.

However, having a genetic mutation associated with Parkinson's does not guarantee the development of the disease. According to the Parkinson's Foundation, even in individuals with such mutations, the likelihood of developing Parkinson's is low. Nonetheless, genetic mutations may significantly contribute to the underlying causes of Parkinson's, prompting extensive research efforts to enhance understanding, improve treatments, and hopefully find a cure.

Environment and Lifestyle

Environmental factors and lifestyle choices may also play a role in causing or increasing the risk of Parkinson's disease. Your occupation, place of residence, and exposure to toxins could potentially contribute to the development of the disease.

While the exact link between environmental factors and Parkinson's disease remains unclear, evidence suggests that certain toxins may play a role in its development. "There are certain toxins that have been shown to increase the risk of Parkinson's," says Dr. Nwabuobi, citing Agent Orange, which many Vietnam veterans were exposed to, as an example. Additionally, exposure to certain metals, herbicides, or fungicides may increase the risk of Parkinson's. Paraquat, in particular, is of concern, despite being banned in many countries.

Researchers are also investigating whether traumatic brain injuries or concussions can cause Parkinson's disease. Studies indicate that even a single concussion can significantly increase the risk of developing Parkinson's disease.

In conclusion, while much remains unknown about the precise causes of Parkinson's disease, ongoing research into genetics, environmental factors, and lifestyle choices offers hope for better understanding, treatment, and ultimately, a cure. Dr. Nwabuobi encourages individuals, especially those with a family history of the disease, to undergo genetic testing to further advance our knowledge in this field.

What are the five phases of Parkinson's disease?

Parkinson's disease presents as a progressive neurological movement disorder, wherein symptoms tend to exacerbate over time. According to the Parkinson's Foundation, individuals typically transition through the stages of the disease gradually, though a sudden worsening of symptoms over days or weeks might suggest other underlying issues. Unlike some medical conditions where a lab test can pinpoint the stage of progression, determining the stage of Parkinson's relies heavily on assessing the severity of motor symptoms and their impact on daily functioning.

While the manifestation of Parkinson's stages may vary among individuals, a general pattern exists, as outlined by the Parkinson's Foundation:

Stage 1:

During the initial phase, individuals may experience mild motor symptoms such as tremors, yet they can still carry out daily activities without significant hindrance. Typically, movement difficulties are confined to one side of the body, accompanied by subtle changes in facial expressions, posture, or gait.

Stage 2:

Symptoms become more pronounced in stage 2, with movement difficulties and muscle stiffness affecting both sides of the body. Routine tasks may become more time-consuming, and individuals might struggle with walking or maintaining proper posture.

Stage 3:

Considered mid-stage Parkinson's, stage 3 marks the onset of balance issues and an increased risk of falls. Daily activities like cooking, cleaning, dressing, and eating may pose greater challenges, although most individuals remain largely independent.

Stage 4:

In this phase, symptoms intensify, necessitating the use of mobility aids such as walkers. Full-time assistance may become necessary for activities of daily living as the disease progresses further.

Stage 5:

This represents the most advanced stage, characterized by severe symptoms. Leg stiffness may hinder standing or walking, potentially confining individuals to a wheelchair or bed. Round-the-clock nursing care becomes essential, with hallucinations and delusions becoming more common.

Clinicians often refer to these stages using the Hoehn and Yahr scale, categorizing stages 1 and 2 as early-stage, stages 2 and 3 as mid-stage, and stages 4 and 5 as late-stage Parkinson's disease.

Here's a breakdown of what occurs at each stage.

Understanding the stages of Parkinson's disease offers a comprehensive framework for individuals grappling with the condition and their healthcare providers, providing invaluable insight into the potential trajectory of the disorder. Parkinson's disease, characterized by its hallmark symptoms including resting tremors, muscular rigidity, and bradykinesia (slowness of movement), presents a complex and multifaceted clinical landscape, wherein no two cases unfold in precisely the same manner.

During the initial stages of Parkinson's disease, individuals may experience relatively mild symptoms that do not significantly disrupt their daily routines or activities. These early manifestations might be subtle and easily overlooked, such as slight tremors or a mild reduction in movement speed. In some cases, individuals may not even realize they have the condition at this stage, attributing their symptoms to other factors or simply dismissing them as signs of aging or fatigue.

However, as Parkinson's disease progresses, its impact on mobility and daily functioning becomes more pronounced and challenging to manage. Individuals may gradually confront a myriad of motor and non-motor symptoms that significantly impede their quality of life. Simple tasks that were once taken for granted, such as walking, standing up from a chair, or even maintaining balance while performing routine activities, may become increasingly arduous.

Over time, the disease's progression can lead to profound and debilitating mobility issues, greatly limiting an individual's independence and ability to engage in activities of daily living. Severe motor complications, such as freezing of gait, dystonia, and dyskinesia, may further exacerbate these challenges, making even basic movements exceedingly difficult to execute.

Furthermore, Parkinson's disease is not solely defined by its physical manifestations; it also exacts a significant toll on cognitive function, emotional well-being, and overall quality of life. Non-motor symptoms such as cognitive impairment, depression, anxiety, sleep disturbances, and autonomic dysfunction can significantly impact an individual's psychological and emotional state, further complicating their journey with the disease.

Navigating the unpredictable course of Parkinson's disease requires a comprehensive understanding of its stages and symptoms, as well as proactive planning and collaboration between patients, caregivers, and healthcare providers. By anticipating the potential challenges and hurdles that lie ahead, individuals can better prepare themselves to cope with the evolving demands of the disease, optimize their treatment strategies, and maintain a sense of control and autonomy in their lives. Additionally, fostering a supportive network of caregivers, friends, and healthcare professionals can provide invaluable emotional and practical support throughout the journey with Parkinson's disease.

At what rate does Parkinson's disease advance?

The progression of Parkinson's disease typically unfolds gradually over the span of years, with individuals often traversing its stages at a slow pace. Studies indicate that the advancement of the disease tends to occur less swiftly in those diagnosed at a younger age, such as in their mid-50s, compared to those diagnosed later in life.

Moreover, Parkinson's disease may initiate decades before any noticeable motor symptoms manifest in a patient. Lynda Nwabuobi, MD, assistant professor of clinical neurology at Weill Cornell Parkinson's Disease and Movement Disorders Institute, underscores this, stating, "We know that Parkinson's disease actually starts many, many years before you see that tremor or that shuffling. We think at least 30 years."

This early phase of Parkinson's disease is termed the "pre-motor" stage, occurring prior to a formal diagnosis, and may encompass symptoms like anosmia (loss of smell), REM sleep behavior disorder (wherein a person acts out their dreams), and constipation.

"Patients will often tell you, 'Yeah, I haven't had a good sense of smell for many, many years,'" notes Dr. Nwabuobi. "Or their spouse says, 'He kicks a lot in his sleep. He's done that since we were married.'"

However, the progression of Parkinson's disease, much like its symptoms, varies from person to person. Dr. Nwabuobi highlights this diversity, saying, "Some people have had Parkinson's for two years and they're not doing so well. And then some people have Parkinson's for 20 years and they're doing great and living their lives."

Thankfully, various treatments exist to assist individuals in managing symptoms and leading more functional lives across the different stages of Parkinson's disease.

"We have a lot of very good medications," adds Dr. Nwabuobi. "I tell people, 'If you're to get a neurodegenerative disease, Parkinson's is not a bad one to have.'"

Chapter 3: How do doctors identify Parkinson's disease?

The process of diagnosing Parkinson's disease extends beyond a mere checklist of symptoms, as it encompasses a nuanced understanding of the interplay between various motor and non-motor manifestations. Dr. Nwabuobi underscores this complexity by highlighting that individuals may present with a diverse array of symptoms, with some experiencing a predominance of non-motor manifestations while others exhibit a greater prominence of motor symptoms. However, amidst this variability, certain hallmark motor symptoms serve as pivotal indicators in the diagnostic process.

During medical evaluations, clinicians meticulously scrutinize for the presence of specific motor symptoms that are indicative of Parkinson's disease. These include rest tremor, bradykinesia (slowness of movement), rigidity (stiffness), and impaired balance. While the manifestation of non-motor symptoms adds layers to the clinical presentation, it's the presence of these motor symptoms that often form the cornerstone of diagnosis.

Moreover, the diagnostic criteria set forth by the Parkinson's Foundation necessitates a sustained observation of motor symptoms over time. It's not merely a matter of sporadic occurrence but rather a consistent manifestation of at least two of the four primary motor symptoms. This requirement underscores the progressive nature of Parkinson's disease, emphasizing the importance of longitudinal assessment to discern its presence conclusively.

By elucidating these diagnostic intricacies, we gain a deeper appreciation for the nuanced approach required in identifying Parkinson's disease. It underscores the necessity for clinicians to carefully consider the constellation of symptoms, both motor and non-motor, while maintaining a vigilant eye on the progression of motor manifestations over time. Such comprehensive evaluation ensures an accurate diagnosis and facilitates the initiation of timely interventions to optimize patient outcomes and quality of life.

What options are available for managing Parkinson's disease?

Regrettably, as of now, Parkinson's disease remains without a definitive cure. Nonetheless, there's reason for optimism as there exist highly efficacious medications aimed at mitigating the symptoms associated with Parkinson's. "I often convey to individuals that if they were to develop a neurodegenerative condition, Parkinson's wouldn't necessarily be the worst one to have because we possess a plethora of commendable medications to address it," remarks Dr. Nwabuobi.

The primary objective of Parkinson's medications revolves around alleviating tremors, rigidity, and bradykinesia. "However, it's imperative to note that none of these medications have demonstrated the capability to decelerate the progression of the disease," advises Dr. Nwabuobi.

Keeping this in consideration, individuals diagnosed with Parkinson's may not immediately require medication if their symptoms are mild and don't significantly impact their quality of life, Dr. Nwabuobi adds. Should medications eventually prove inadequate in managing Parkinson's symptoms, surgical interventions like deep brain stimulation might emerge as a viable option. This procedure involves implanting a device that emits electrical signals to the brain regions responsible for motor function.

Nonetheless, medications and surgery aren't the exclusive avenues for addressing Parkinson's symptoms. Lifestyle modifications, particularly aerobic exercise, can also yield significant benefits. Dr. Nwabuobi recommends that individuals with Parkinson's engage in 30 minutes of exercise daily, five days a week. "It's the one aspect where we have some evidence suggesting it may slow the progression of the disease," she notes. "I can discern which of my patients are exercising and which are not. You can observe the fluidity in their movements. They feel better and they appear better."

Treatment and manifestations of Parkinson's disease.

Certain medications, particularly those that inhibit the action of dopamine, can potentially induce symptoms akin to Parkinson's disease. This condition, termed drug-induced parkinsonism, though distinct from Parkinson's itself, may closely resemble its symptoms. Among the medications implicated in causing Parkinson's-like symptoms are antipsychotics such as fluphenazine, pimozide, haloperidol, and perphenazine, as well as anti-nausea medications like chlorpromazine, droperidol, and promethazine. Additionally, drugs used to treat hyperkinetic movement disorders, including tetrabenazine, deutetrabenazine, and valbenazine, have been associated with similar effects.

It's essential to note that while these medications and others might trigger symptoms resembling

Parkinson's, they do not directly cause the disease. Typically, the symptoms tend to dissipate within hours or days upon discontinuation of the offending medication, according to the Parkinson's Disease Society. However, in some instances, Parkinsonian symptoms persist even after cessation of the medication, eventually leading to a diagnosis of Parkinson's disease.

Researchers posit that in such cases, the medication itself may not be the direct cause of Parkinson's, but rather, it could have unveiled an underlying depletion of dopamine levels in affected individuals. In essence, the medication acted as the proverbial "straw that broke the camel's back," as suggested by the American Parkinson Disease Association.

Ongoing research into the etiology of Parkinson's disease continues to expand. If you experience symptoms suggestive of Parkinson's, such as hand tremors, bradykinesia, postural instability, or changes in speech or handwriting, it's crucial to consult with a healthcare professional for proper diagnosis and management.

Chapter 4: Guide to Diet and Nutrition for Parkinson's Disease

Parkinson's disease, a neurodegenerative condition, is not selective—it can manifest in individuals from various walks of life. Each year, around 50,000 people in the United States are confronted with the diagnosis of Parkinson's disease, marking the beginning of a journey fraught with challenges and uncertainties. However, amidst these uncertainties, one avenue that holds promise in potentially mitigating the onset or progression of Parkinson's lies in the realm of dietary choices.

Emerging research and expert opinions increasingly suggest that maintaining a healthful diet could serve as a valuable adjunct to conventional treatments for Parkinson's disease. By making deliberate choices about what we consume, we might be able to tip the scales in favor of better health outcomes. Indeed, a well-rounded diet not only nourishes the body but also nurtures the mind and spirit, fostering resilience in the face of neurological challenges.

Moreover, beyond the realm of prevention, there's mounting evidence that dietary interventions could play a significant role in slowing down the progression of Parkinson's disease and alleviating its symptoms. This perspective underscores the profound connection between nutrition and neurological health—a connection that has the potential to redefine how we approach the management of chronic conditions like Parkinson's.

With this in mind, it becomes imperative to explore the intricacies of a Parkinson's-friendly diet—a dietary framework specifically designed to address the unique nutritional needs and challenges faced by individuals living with Parkinson's disease. By delving into expert recommendations and evidence-based strategies, we can unravel the nuances of crafting a menu that not only supports overall well-being but also empowers individuals to take an active role in managing their health.

In essence, the journey toward a healthier life with Parkinson's disease begins at the dinner table, where every morsel we choose has the potential to shape our future trajectory. Through informed choices and a commitment to nourishing our bodies with wholesome, nutrient-rich foods, we can embark on a path of empowerment and resilience in the face of Parkinson's disease.

Essential Foods for the Parkinson's Diet

Researchers are placing significant emphasis on exploring dietary approaches that have the potential to alleviate the symptoms associated with Parkinson's disease. The concept of "good food" extends beyond merely providing essential vitamins and minerals; it encompasses fostering overall health and safeguarding against detrimental environmental factors.

One crucial area of focus is antioxidants. Oxidative stress, triggered by free-floating elements like pollution, cigarette smoke, and household cleaners, can contribute to cell damage and the progression of nerve cell death in Parkinson's disease. Professionals such as Jelena Etemovic from Cedars-Sinai advocate for a diet rich in plant-based foods abundant in antioxidants to counteract oxidative stress.

Examples of antioxidants include vitamins A, E, and C, which are found abundantly in various foods such as berries (including blueberries, strawberries, raspberries, and cherries), cruciferous vegetables (like broccoli, cauliflower, Brussels sprouts, and kale), nightshade vegetables (such as tomatoes, eggplant, and peppers), spices (including turmeric, cinnamon, and ginger), and tree nuts (such as walnuts, Brazil nuts, pecans, and pistachios).

Another crucial dietary component for individuals with Parkinson's disease is healthy fats. Neuroinflammation, characterized by inflammation of the nervous system, is linked to accelerated nerve damage in PD. Healthy fats act as anti-inflammatory agents, potentially reducing neuroinflammation and slowing the progression of the disease. Omega-3 fatty acids, essential for a balanced diet, can be obtained from sources like fish (such as salmon, mackerel, cod, herring, and lake trout), nuts (particularly walnuts), seeds (including flaxseeds, chia seeds, pumpkin seeds), and soybeans. Supplements like fish oil, flaxseed oil, cod liver oil, and algae oil are also available, although whole foods are generally preferred.

Furthermore, a variety of other healthy fats can be incorporated into the diet, including healthy oils (like olive oil, coconut oil, and avocado oil), avocados, nut butters (such as almond butter and peanut butter), and eggs. However, it's advisable to be cautious with egg yolks due to their high saturated fat content, opting for egg whites whenever possible.

Opting for high-quality foods, such as organic produce and sustainably sourced animal products, can minimize exposure to toxins like pesticides, herbicides, and GMOs commonly found in conventional food products. While organic options may be more expensive, selecting local and in-season varieties can help accommodate budgetary constraints.

When purchasing and preparing meat and animal products, prioritize high-quality options such as grass-fed beef (preferably organic), free-range eggs (preferably organic), organic milk and dairy products (in moderation), wild-caught seafood, and free-range chicken and turkey (preferably organic). Choosing animal products from animals raised on cleaner and healthier diets is optimal since you essentially consume what the animal consumes.

Additionally, consuming foods rich in flavonoids may offer benefits for individuals with Parkinson's disease. Flavonoids, antioxidant compounds abundant in brightly colored foods like blueberries, dark chocolate, tea, strawberries, and red wine, have been associated with potentially reducing mortality rates among Parkinson's patients. However, it's essential to consume alcoholic beverages like red wine in moderation, as excessive alcohol intake can lead to empty calories, nutrient deficiencies, accidents, and unrelated health issues.

Steer clear of these foods when following a Parkinson's dietary plan.

Scholars and medical professionals have increasingly turned their attention to exploring dietary interventions that could potentially alleviate the symptoms associated with Parkinson's disease. They emphasize the significance of a wholesome diet not only in providing essential nutrients but also in fostering overall well-being and shielding against detrimental environmental influences.

One crucial aspect of dietary strategies involves the incorporation of antioxidants. Oxidative stress, triggered by various environmental pollutants such as smoke and toxins, has been implicated in the degeneration of nerve cells characteristic of Parkinson's disease. Consequently, researchers like Jelena Etemovic of Cedars-Sinai advocate for the consumption of antioxidant-rich foods to counteract oxidative stress. These foods, abundant in vitamins A, E, and C, encompass a diverse array of options including berries, cruciferous vegetables, nightshade vegetables, spices like turmeric and ginger, as well as tree nuts.

Moreover, dietary choices can also modulate inflammation, a process closely linked to accelerated nerve damage in Parkinson's. Healthy fats serve as potent anti-inflammatory agents, potentially attenuating neuroinflammation and slowing disease progression. Omega-3 fatty acids, renowned for their myriad health benefits, are found abundantly in fish, nuts, seeds, and soybeans. While supplements are available, experts recommend obtaining these nutrients from whole foods whenever feasible.

In addition to Omega-3s, other sources of healthy fats merit attention. Foods such as avocados, olive oil, coconut oil, and nut butters provide alternative avenues for incorporating these beneficial fats into the diet. However, caution is advised regarding saturated fats, emphasizing the importance of making prudent choices such as opting for lean meats and minimizing consumption of egg yolks.

Furthermore, the quality of food matters significantly in mitigating exposure to toxins commonly found in conventional produce. Choosing organic options, particularly for fruits, vegetables, and animal products, can help minimize exposure to pesticides, herbicides, and genetically modified organisms (GMOs). While organic foods may incur higher costs, selecting local and seasonal produce can mitigate budgetary constraints.

Furthermore, emerging research highlights the potential benefits of flavonoid-rich foods in managing Parkinson's disease. Flavonoids, abundant in colorful fruits, vegetables, and beverages like tea and red wine, possess antioxidant properties that may confer neuroprotective effects. However, moderation is advised, especially in the case of alcoholic beverages, due to their potential adverse effects and limited nutritional value.

In essence, adopting a dietary regimen rich in antioxidants, healthy fats, and high-quality foods while minimizing exposure to toxins represents a multifaceted approach to supporting overall health and potentially ameliorating the symptoms of Parkinson's disease.

Maintain a Healthy and Balanced Meal Plan

- Crafting a well-rounded dietary regimen with an abundance of fresh vegetables and fruits laid out on your table is not just about the act of eating; it's a proactive measure in mitigating the progression of Parkinson's disease. However, achieving this goal requires more than just eliminating certain foods from your diet; it necessitates embracing a holistic approach to healthy living to bolster your defenses against the debilitating effects of the disease. Here are some comprehensive diet and nutrition recommendations to steer you toward maintaining optimal health:

-

- 1. Prioritize Balanced, Timely Meals: Instead of fixating on restrictive eating habits, embrace a diverse array of foods from all essential food groups, including fruits, vegetables, grains, protein sources, and a moderate intake of dairy. Furthermore, maintaining regular meal times, ensuring you don't skip meals, and refraining from prolonged periods without eating (more than 4 hours) are crucial strategies to prevent weight loss and optimize the absorption and utilization of nutrients.

*

* 2. Avoid Fad Diets: Resist the allure of trendy diets that promise quick fixes. Unless a certified health professional tailors a menu based on a specific diet to suit your individual needs, it's advisable to approach such diets with caution. Always consult your healthcare provider before embarking on any new or trending diet plan.

-

- 3. Limit Intake of Sweet and Salty Foods: Reducing consumption of foods high in sugar and sodium is essential. Sweet treats, particularly baked goods and desserts, often pack a caloric punch without offering substantial nutritional benefits. Excessive sugar intake can lead to weight gain, elevated blood sugar levels, and dental issues.

-

- In addition to these dietary guidelines, there are specific dietary habits that can help alleviate Parkinson's symptoms and support overall well-being:

-

- - Increase Fiber Intake and Hydration: Combat constipation, a common symptom of Parkinson's, by consuming adequate fiber from whole grains, fresh fruits, and leafy greens. Hydration is equally important; drinking plenty of water not only aids digestion but also helps metabolize prescription medications effectively.

-

- - Incorporate Fava Beans: Fava beans naturally contain levodopa, an amino acid that mimics the effects of commonly prescribed medications for Parkinson's disease.

-

- - Opt for Berries as Healthy Snacks: Keep a supply of berries on hand to satisfy cravings for sweets. Natural sugars found in berries offer a healthier alternative to processed sugars and are rich in essential vitamins and minerals.

-

- Ultimately, maintaining a diet rich in nutrient-dense foods and adhering to a regular eating schedule is key. Avoid foods that may adversely affect blood pressure, heart health, and saturated fat intake. Planning meals in advance can help alleviate uncertainty about what to eat, ensuring that your dietary choices align with your health goals. If you're unsure about dietary recommendations, seek guidance from healthcare professionals who can provide personalized advice tailored to your specific needs in managing Parkinson's disease.

Chapter 5: Nutritious, Tasty Recipes for Parkinson's disease

Mushroom and kidney bean pattie

Ingredients

1 medium sweet potato

2 large Portobello/Field mushrooms

Extra virgin olive oil

1 cup of cooked kidney beans

1 small carrot, roughly chopped

1/4 medium onion, roughly chopped

1 bunch fresh coriander, roughly chopped

Breadcrumbs

1 teaspoon fresh chili (optional)

1 teaspoon ground cumin

1 egg

Salad to serve (sliced tomato, lettuce leaves)

Preparation

Peel and cut the sweet potato into battens or chips 2cm x 8cm. Place on a baking tray with non-stick paper.

Remove mushroom stalks, place on the same baking tray and drizzle with extra virgin olive oil.

Roast in a 200ºC (392ºF) oven for 20 minutes, or until mushrooms and sweet potato are cooked.

In a food processor combine kidney beans, carrot, onion, coriander, breadcrumbs and spices. Process to a rough paste. Transfer to a bowl and mix through the egg. Form into 2 patties.

Fry the patties in extra virgin olive oil until warmed through and browned on the outside.

To assemble, place the salad on the bottom of the plate, then the patty, your favourite sauce or chutney and top with the roasted mushroom. Serve with the sweet potato chips on the side

Lentil and Vegetable Penne pasta

Ingredients

2 tablespoons extra virgin olive oil

3 small carrots, peeled, finely chopped

3 celery sticks, finely chopped

2 garlic cloves, thinly chopped

1 large brown onion, coarsely chopped

1 small red capsicum, finely chopped

10-12 button mushrooms, thinly chopped

225 grams cooked brown lentils

150 grams Passata

500 grams No added sugar pasta sauce

500 grams High fibre pasta Penne

Preparation

Heat the extra virgin olive oil in a large heavy-based saucepan over medium heat.

Add celery, carrot, onion, garlic and cook until just tender.

Add lentils, capsicum and mushrooms and cook, until just tender.

Egg and vegetable muffins

Ingredients

4 eggs

15-20 spinach leaves, roughly chopped

¼ cup red capsicum, finely diced

¼ cup corn cornels (cooked)

6 cherry tomatoes (cut into quarters)

Preparation

Preheat the oven to 190°C/375°F.

Grease a 6-cup muffin tin or use paper cupcake cases.

Crack the eggs into a bowl and whisk together with a fork.

Add the capsicum, spinach, tomato and corn to the whisked eggs and stir.

Pour the egg mixture into the greased 6-cup muffin tin or paper cupcake cases.

Bake for 10-12 minutes or until eggs are set.

Allow to cool for 5 minutes before removing from muffin tin.

Beetroot and cashew puree

Ingredients

250 grams fresh Beetroot

60 grams unsalted Cashews

Extra virgin Olive Oil

Salt

Pepper

Equipment

Steamer

Stick blender with chopper attachment or a food

processor

Sieve

Spoon

Preparation

Place whole beetroots into the bottom level of a bench top or cooktop steamer. Place cashews in the steaming basket above and cook until beetroot is tender.

Remove beetroot skins and place into the stick blender chopper/food processor along with the steamed cashews, salt and pepper & a drizzle of olive oil then blitz until smooth. Note– when blitzing, stop regularly to scrape down the sides of the processor or chopping attachment, drizzle more olive oil if mixture appears too dry.

Pass mixture through a sieve to ensure all hard, grainy particles are removed.

Using a touch of lemon infused olive oil works very well in this recipe if you have it available.

Roast pumpkin puree

Ingredients

500 grams butternut pumpkin

Extra virgin olive oil

Salt

Pepper

Equipment

Baking Dish

Stick blender

Jug or beaker

Preparation

Chop pumpkin, removing skin and seeds, and
place in a baking dish.

Drizzle with extra virgin olive oil, sprinkle of salt and pepper and place into the oven.

Once tender remove from the oven and transfer into a jug/beaker.

Use stick blender to puree until smooth.

Carrot & Miso Soup with Silken Tofu

Ingredients

1 kg Carrots Peeled & Chopped

1 large Onion Diced

1.5 tsp Grated Fresh Ginger

3 cloves Garlic Crushed

1 litre Vegetable Stock

4 tbsp White Miso

200gm Silken Tofu

2 tbsp Sesame Oil

Salt

Pepper

Coconut cream & additional sesame oil for garnishing (or extra virgin olive oil)

Equipment

Blender or Stick Blender

Preparation

Sauté onions, garlic, ginger and carrots in sesame oil until onions are translucent. Add in vegetable stock, cover and simmer for 30 minutes stirring occasionally.

Add in white miso and silken tofu and blend using your modification tool of choice, adding more stock or water as needed (or alternatively coconut cream.) Add salt and pepper to taste.

Chocolate smoothie recipes

Ingredients

150 ml unsweetened almond milk

½ avocado

4 fresh strawberries

1 teaspoon raw cacao powder

1½ teaspoon natvia (natural sweetener)

Ice to serve

Preparation

Combine almond milk, avocado flesh, strawberries, cacao and natvia in a blender.

Blend until smooth.

Serve in a glass with ice.

Estimated nutrition information per serving: 203 calories, 3.6 grams protein, 18.5 grams fat, 4.7 grams carbohydrate, 65 mg sodium

Choc Coconut Smoothie

Ingredients

90ml coconut milk

90ml water

1 teaspoon raw cacao powder

1 teaspoon natvia (natural sweetener)

Ice to serve

Preparation

Combine coconut milk, water, cacao and natvia in a blender.

Blend until smooth.

Serve in a glass with ice.

Mango Smothie

Ingredients

1 medium Mango

170 ml coconut milk

100 ml coconut water

5-10 ice cubes (optional)

Preparation

Peel the mango and slice the flesh and add to the blender. Then add coconut milk, coconut water and ice if desired.

Blend until smooth.

Serve in a glass.

Berry smoothie with blueberries & strawberries

Ingredients

200 ml coconut water

1/2 cup strawberries

1/2 cup blueberries

1/2 cup coconut yoghurt

Preparation

In a blender, combine all ingredients and blend until smooth.
Serve in a glass.

Banana Oat and Cinnamon Smoothie

Ingredients

1 medium banana

250 ml oat milk

½ teaspoon ground cinnamon

½ teaspoon honey (optional)

Preparation

Peel the banana and break into pieces and add to the blender. Then add oat milk, cinnamon and honey if desired.

Blend until smooth.

Serve in a glass.

Chocolate avocado mousse

Ingredients

2 large avocados

3 tbsp honey

1 tsp vanilla bean extract

40 grams cocoa powder

Preparation

Place avocado flesh into a food processor with the honey, vanilla bean extract and cacao powder.

Blend/process until silky and smooth.

Transfer into chosen serving dish/es and refrigerate for at least 1 hour before serving.

Thai fishcakes with zingy salsa

Ingredients

150-200g white fish

4 spring onions, chopped

1 inch fresh root ginger, grated

1 tsp Thai green curry paste

1 egg, beaten

2 tbsp chopped coriander

1 tbsp flour

Juice and zest of a lime

Black pepper

1 tsp coconut oil

Preparation

Finely chop the fish and place in a large bowl with the spring onions, ginger, curry paste, fish sauce, egg and coriander.

Mix well and then stir in the flour, lime juice and zest and season with black pepper. The mixture may be a bit wet at this stage. You can add a bit more flour if you like.

Divide into four generous portions. Put a little flour on your hands and form each portion into a ball. Flatten slightly and fry in the coconut oil for five to eight minutes until golden brown and cooked through.

Serve with a green salad or my zingy salsa.

Cinnamon nectarines with vanilla scented yoghurt by Jane McClenaghan

Ingredients

1-2 tsp agave syrup

2 nectarines, halved with stone removed

½-1 tsp ground cinnamon

½ vanilla pod

2 tbsp Greek yoghurt

Preparation

Preheat your oven to 180C/350F/Gas 4.

Drizzle a little agave syrup over each nectarine half and sprinkle with cinnamon. Cover with tinfoil and bake for 15-20 minutes until soft.

Slice the vanilla pod lengthways and, with the tip of a sharp knife, scrape out the seeds and stir into the Greek yoghurt.

Serve the nectarines hot or cold with a drizzle of agave syrup and a dollop of the vanilla scented Greek yoghurt.

Salmon fillet marinated in lime juice with aniseed and cabbage salads

Ingredients

500g salmon fillet

100ml lime juice

2 tbsp raisins

2 tbsp white wine or cider vinegar

2 tbsp red wine or raspberry vinegar

200g white cabbage

200g red cabbage

2 tbsp sunflower oil

1 tbsp fresh tarragon (chopped)

1 tbsp aniseed

1/3 tsp cayenne pepper

Salt

Sunflower oil

Preparation

Start your preparations for this dish at least four hours before serving. Start your preparations for the salads a day before serving.

Cut the salmon into equal slices, each 2cm thick (approx.).

Sprinkle salt, aniseed and hot pepper on both sides slices and leave in the fridge to rest for 30 minutes.

Dressing

Place the marinated slices into the lime juice for 90 minutes on each side.

Mix the lime juice with the sunflower oil and the tarragon into the dressing.

Salads

Put two tablespoons of raisins in vinegar, leave for two hours.

Add to the sliced cabbages.

Add salt and freshly ground black pepper, oil and tarragon.

Place the salads in two parallel lines in the middle of a plate.

Place the salmon slices on top and sprinkle with the dressing.

Porcini enriched poultry broth with ravioli filled with chicken and/or mushrooms

Ingredients

2 chopped of sunflower oil

1kg chicken wings

200g mixed small vegetables

2 celery ribs with leaves

2 medium carrots

2 onions

1 leek

100g dried porcini mushrooms

2 cloves

4 bay leaves

6 peppercorns (whole)

12 Chinese ravioli leaves

250g mushrooms

1 tbsp flour

1 tbsp chives or sage

1 egg yolk mixed with 1 tsp oil

Preparation

Start your preparations for this broth a day before serving.

Heat the sunflower oil in a pan.

Add the chicken and vegetables and sauté until brown.

Add 1 litre of cold water and the porcini.

Slowly bring to a boil.

Simmer for at least four hours.

Take out the chicken, vegetables and porcini.

Remove meat from the bones.

Rinse and chop the porcini.

Refrigerate the broth for eight hours overnight, skim fat from the surface.

Chop the mushrooms and fry in oil.

On a low heat, add porcini, chicken meat, flour and 2 tbsp water.

Cook for five minutes, refrigerate and chop fine in your KitchenAid.

Mix in the herbs.

Brush egg yolk with oil onto each pastry leaf.

Place a teaspoonful of the mushroom mix on the corner of each leaf and fold into a triangle.

Poach for five minutes in broth.

Pulled wild boar or venison stewed in dark ale with plums, mashed potatoes, parsnip and broccoli

Ingredients

800g stewing venison or boar (large chunks)

2 tbsp sunflower oil

1 tbsp crushed juniper berries

1 tsp rosemary leaves

1 tbsp chopped thyme leaves

2 tbsp of flour

5 bay leaves

1 bottle brown ale

1 tbsp of red wine vinegar

12 prunes

Parsnips (as much as you like)

Broccoli (as much as you like)

Preparation

Start your preparations for this stew a day before serving it.

Mix juniper berries, rosemary, thyme leaves and flour with some black pepper and salt.

Toss your meat through this mix and press until well coated.

Heat the oil in a large pan at a high temperature.

Fry the meat on all sides to brown.

Add bay leaves, ale, vinegar and some water to cover the meat.

Cook on a very low fire until your meat falls apart.

Take the meat out and refrigerate; pull into strips.

Reduce the liquid left in the pan on a high fire until 250ml (approx.) is left.

Put the pulled meat in the sauce, add the prunes.

Fry the parsnip in sunflower oil.

Heat the broccoli in your microwave.

Put the parsnip in the middle of a plate and arrange the meat over it.

Arrange broccoli around the meat.

Winter trifle; chestnut purée and cottage cheese, apple, chopped amarena cherries and oatmeal cookies

Ingredients

300g Sweet chestnut purée

250g cottage cheese

1 teaspoon vanilla sugar

1 apple (finely diced)

200g amarena cherries (finely chopped)

120g crumbled oat cookies

Amaretto liqueur

Homemade custard

Preparation

Poach the diced apple for two minutes in hot water with some sugar.

Mix together the chestnut purée, cottage cheese and vanilla sugar.

Build your trifle in layers in a large glass bowl or in a separate glass for each guest.

Vegetarian 'Beet Wellington' with mushrooms, aubergines and garlic

Ingredients

140g fresh, organic beetroots

100g mushrooms

4 sheets 20x20cm puff pastry

3 tbsp breadcrumbs

2 shallots (roughly chopped)

2 pinches of aniseed

1 clove of garlic (roughly chopped)

1 tbsp of cut sage

1 tbsp tomato purée

1 aubergine (diced)

1 egg yolk (mixed with 1 tbsp oil and water)

1 tsp poppy seeds (optional)

Sunflower oil

Flour

Pepper

Salt (optional)

Preparation

Preheat oven to 180°C.

Place the beetroots into an oven dish and brush them with sunflower oil.

Roast the beetroots in the oven for 45 minutes.

Remove the skin from the beetroots.

Mix sunflower oil with pepper, 1 pinch of aniseed and sage.

Brush the oil mixture onto the beetroots. Sprinkle some salt on top (optional).

Heat sunflower oil in a frying pan and fry the aubergine, shallots, garlic and mushrooms.

Add the tomato purée and a splash of water, stir thoroughly.

Add the breadcrumbs, sage and 1 pinch of aniseed.

Cook on a low heat for ten minutes, stirring from time to time.

Purée the mixture in a blender, leave to cool.

Pre-heat the oven to 220°C.

Place sheets of pastry on a cool, floured surface.

Brush the edges of the pastry with the mixture of egg yolk, water and oil.

Place ½ tbsp of breadcrumbs in the middle of each sheet.

Spread the purée mixture over the sheets of pastry.

Place the beetroot on top of the purée mixture.

As tightly as possible, fold the pastry sheets over the purée and beetroot.

Turn the pastry over and brush egg yolk over the top.

Sprinkle poppy seeds over the dough (optional).

Bake the Beet Wellington for 20 minutes, until golden brown.

Colourful broccoli, shiitake mushrooms and cashew nut stir-fry

Ingredients

2 eggs

300g broccoli florets

240g thin Chinese egg noodles (boiled)

200g baby corn cobs

100g shiitake mushrooms

100g cashew nuts (coarsely chopped)

4 tbsp oil

2 tbsp water

2 tbsp ginger syrup

2 tbsp lemon juice

2 tbsp sunflower oil

1 tbsp sesame oil

2 cloves of garlic (thinly sliced)

1 red onion, sliced into rings

Preparation

Remove the stalks from the shiitakes and cut the tops into quarters.

Blanch the baby corn for two minutes and then the broccoli for one minute.

Fry both the onion and garlic in a wok.

Add the shiitake mushrooms and fry for one minute on a high heat.

Add the baby corn and broccoli.

Add the water, ginger syrup and lemon juice. Heat for a further two minutes.

Add the nuts.

Fry the egg noodles in a mixture of sunflower and sesame oil.

Beat the eggs and stir into the noodles.

Rich chocolate fondue with strawberries and pineapple

Ingredients

300g pure chocolate (70% cocoa)

250g washed strawberries

250g fresh pineapple, diced and dried

100ml whipped cream

4 slices of cake

Preparation

Warm the chocolate with the cream in a bowl, using the bain-marie method, while stirring into a smooth sauce.

Place a fondue hot plate on the table and light the candle below. Put the pan with chocolate sauce on top of the plate.

Skewer a piece of fruit on a fork and dip into the chocolate sauce.

Bread rosettes with spinach, feta and oregano

Ingredients

500g whole wheat flour

500g spinach leaves

200g crumbled feta

20g fresh or 2 packets of dry yeast

2 tsp dried oregano

2 tbsp olive oil

250ml water (lukewarm)

2 cloves of garlic (coarsely chopped)

4 tbsp olive oil

pinch of salt

Preparation

Put the flour in a mixing bowl. Add the fresh, crumbled yeast or dried yeast and mix through the flour.

Mix in 1 tsp of oregano. Make a well in the centre and pour in the olive oil and water. Mix until a soft dough forms. Add the salt. Leave to rest for 15 minutes.

Knead the dough for 5–10 minutes until supple and elastic.

Form a ball, place it in the mixing bowl, cover with cling film and allow to rise in a warm spot for 1 hour, or until the volume has doubled.

Fry the garlic in olive oil at low heat until glazed. Turn the heat up and add the spinach. Allow to cook and turn over from time to time.

Use a strainer to remove all the water from the spinach.

Apply olive oil to the work surface.

Roll the dough into a 50 x 30cm rectangle with a thickness of 0.75cm.

Divide the spinach and feta over the dough.

Make a loose roll, starting at a short side.

Cut the roll of dough into 12 slices and place the slices on a baking tray covered with baking paper.

Cover with a floured towel and allow to rise for 1 hour.

Pre-heat the oven at 200°C and bake the bread in 20–25 minutes until golden brown.

Allow the bread to cool on a grid outside the oven.

Sicilian caponata: aubergines in a 'puttanesca' tomato sauce

Ingredients

2 aubergines (diced)

2 onions (coarsely chopped)

3 celery stalks (peeled and diced)

3 tbsp olive oil

2 plum tomatoes (finely chopped)

2 cloves of garlic (thin slices)

3 celery stalks (peeled and diced)

2 beefsteak tomatoes (diced)

1 red bell pepper (finely chopped)

12 black, pitted olives (coarsely chopped)

2 tbsp green herbs

2 tbsp jam sugar

1 tbsp white wine vinegar

½ tbsp small capers

1 tsp paprika

cayenne pepper

salt and pepper

Preparation

Sicilian Caponata

Place the diced aubergine into salted cold water for 10 minutes.

Gently dry the diced aubergine.

Fry the aubergine with the onion in olive oil.

Add the garlic and the celery and braise for 3 minutes.

Add the tomatoes, olives, capers and the sugar.

Deglaze with white wine vinegar.

Season with salt, pepper and cayenne pepper.

Leave to cool and mix in the green herbs.

Putanesca sauce

Fry the onion and bell pepper in olive oil.

Add the tomatoes.

Season with salt, pepper and paprika.

Allow the ingredients to cook thoroughly.

Add water if the sauce becomes too thick.

Pass the sauce through a sieve and leave to cool

Indonesian minced pork with caramelised pumpkin and cucumber soup

Ingredients

Stewed pumpkin with egg

240g brown wholegrain rice

400g pumpkin

400g pork mince

4 eggs

2 tbsp soy sauce

1 tbsp honey or agave syrup

100ml olive oil

4 cloves garlic

fresh ginger (a small piece)

Cucumber soup

 2 cucumbers (large)

1 chicken or vegetable stock

2 onions

salt and pepper

fresh coriander or parsley

Preparation

Peel the cucumbers and cut into chunks. Remove
the seeds from the pumpkin and dice.

Peel the onion and cut into slices.

Peel the ginger and cut into medium-sized chunks.

Mix the garlic and the ginger into the olive oil –
this mixture will form the base of the stew.

Boil the rice and leave to drain.

Preparation: cucumber soup

Fry the onion in a medium-sized saucepan in two tablespoons of the olive oil mixture.

Add the chicken stock and bring to the boil.

Add the cucumber and mix well.

Season with salt and pepper.

Preparation: stewed pumpkin with egg

Soft boil the eggs.

Fry the pumpkin cubes and the pork mince in a pan in two tablespoons of the olive oil mixture.

Add the honey and gently caramelise.

Add the soy sauce and stew until cooked.

Salmon and vegetable potato topper

Ingredients

350ml milk or milk alternative

230g thinly sliced carrots, cooked and drained

230g canned salmon, drained

90g grated Cheddar cheese or vegan cheese

4 tbsp minced onion

4 tbsp minced bell peppers

2 tbsp unsalted butter

1 1/2 tbsp whole wheat flour

1/4 teaspoon garlic powder

1/8 teaspoon ground thyme

ground marjoram

pre-baked potatoes

Preparation

In a medium-sized saucepan, sauté the onion and bell peppers in butter for five minutes or until vegetables are tender.

Combine the flour, garlic powder, thyme and marjoram. Stir into onion mixture. Heat and stir for one or two minutes.

Remove from heat. Slowly stir in the milk or milk alternative.

Return to heat and stir until the sauce becomes thickened and reaches the boil.

Stir in the cheese, cooked carrots and salmon and heat through.

Split the baked potatoes and fluff the insides with a fork. Discard the potato skins.

Spoon the salmon mixture over potatoes and stir lightly to blend with and moisten the potato.

Greek-inspired courgette and aubergine vegetarian moussaka

Ingredients

1kg firm potatoes

30g soy butter

40g wheat flour

700ml unsweetened soy milk

500g tofu (or seitan)

8 fresh tomatoes (or 1 tin of tomatoes)

3 garlic cloves

1 aubergine

1 courgette

1 sweet pepper

1 onion

1 tsp oregano

nutmeg

salt and pepper

olive oil

Preparation

Preheat the oven to 180°C.

Boil the potatoes until 'al dente' and cut into slices.

Slice the aubergine, courgette and sweet pepper.

Dice the tomato.

For the white sauce: melt the soy butter and mix with the flour. Stir well with a wooden ladle until the roux is dry.

Pour the soy milk into the sauce little by little, while stirring with a whisk until it becomes a smooth, firm sauce. NB: you could also bind the soy milk with a white sauce binding agent.

Season with salt, pepper and nutmeg and boil for a few more minutes while stirring.

For the tomato sauce, fry the onions in heated olive oil until glazed.

Add the tofu or seitan and stew for another five minutes on a low heat.

Add oregano, garlic and tomato, bring to the boil while stirring, leave to simmer for 10 minutes.

Place the aubergine, courgettes and the sweet pepper onto a greased oven dish and put into the oven. NB: you could also fry the vegetables on both sides in a pan with olive oil.

Taste tip

Tofu is a meat replacement made of soy milk. It has a bland flavour but easily takes up the flavours of other foods. It is low in fat and rich in proteins. When cut it into cubes, tofu is easy to shallow fry, deep fry and grill. Seitan is a wheat gluten meat replacement.

Finishing

Put a layer of vegetables into a lightly greased deep oven dish. Next, add a layer of potatoes and a layer of tomato sauce.

Finish with the white sauce.

Put the moussaka into the oven for another 15 minutes.

Broccoli and salmon crustless quiche

Ingredients

400g broccoli florets (fresh or frozen)

400g smoked salmon

3ml cream or soy cream

50g grated Emmental cheese

3 eggs

1 extra yolk

1 tbsp dill

salt and pepper

cayenne pepper

nutmeg

Preparation

Break the broccoli into florets, cut the salmon into fine strips, and chop the dill.

Preheat the oven to 180 °C.

Cook the broccoli in lightly salted water, pour into a sieve and rinse immediately in cold running water to preserve its dark green colour. Drain well.

Mix the cream, eggs and herbs, spices and seasoning.

Finely chop the broccoli florets.

Grease or line a baking mould.

Spread the broccoli on the bottom of the tin with a layer of salmon strips on the top.

Fill the moulds three-quarters with the cream mixture.

Sprinkle with grated cheese.

Bake for 25 minutes at 180°C.

Leave the quiche on a cooling rack. Once cool, take the moulds away and put on a plate.

Ground game granny's style: stewed rabbit with plums

Ingredients

4 legs of rabbit or 1 whole rabbit

400g chicory

300g dried plums

30g brown sugar

25g butter

4 onions

3 slices brown bread

3 tbsp grain mustard

2 bottles of beer

2 sprigs thyme

2 bay leaves

1 tbsp vegetable stock

1 tsp wine vinegar

1 lemon

salt and pepper

Preparation

Peel the onion and slice into halved rings.

Remove the outer leaves and the core of the chicory.

Cut the chicory into fine strips and add lemon juice to prevent discolouration.

Soak the plums in cold water.

Season the rabbit with salt and pepper and stew in butter until all sides have browned.

Add the sliced onion, bay leaves and thyme – stew until glazed.

Spread the slices of bread with the grain mustard.

Deglaze with the beer and add the bread slices.

Add stock (and/or water) until the rabbit is just covered.

Add the vinegar and sugar. Leave to simmer for about 30 minutes, until the rabbit is tender.

Add the plums.

Take all the solid ingredients out of the stewing pot, remove thyme and bay leaves and bind the sauce to the required consistency level with the brown sauce binder.

Season with pepper and salt and put everything together again.

Serve.

Chicory with ham and cheese sauce

Ingredients

600g potatoes

200g gruyere cheese (grated)

50g parmesan cheese (grated)

700ml semi-skimmed milk

8 chicory heads (ground)

8 slices cooked ham

50g butter

40g flour

1/2 lemon

1 tsp white sugar

salt and pepper

nutmeg

Preparation

Clean the chicory, remove the outer leaves and the
hard core.

Cut the chicory into fine rings.

Peel and cut the potatoes for the purée.

Roll up the slices of ham and cut them finely.

Stew the chicory in 20g of butter with sugar, salt, pepper and nutmeg until cooked. Leave to drain and reserve the cooking liquid.

Boil the potatoes, mash and season with salt, pepper and nutmeg.

Prepare a béchamel sauce with a roux made from 30g butter and 40g flour. Deglaze the roux with the cold milk and stir firmly with a whisk to prevent clotting.

Tip

You can also prepare the sauce with a white sauce binder.

Season with the preserved cooking liquid of the chicory, pepper, salt and nutmeg.

Finishing

Add ¾ of the cheese to the béchamel sauce and the juice of half a lemon.

Lightly butter a casserole dish.

First put the puree in, then the chicory, on top the ham and finally the cheese sauce.

Sprinkle the remainder of the grated cheese over the top and gratinate under the grill.

Garnish with slices of lemon.

Rich roast pork Orloff with vegetables and red pesto

Ingredients

600g pork (boneless ribs)

6 slices of cooked ham

200g grated cheese (Emmental or Gruèyre)

500ml brown cream sauce

200g mushrooms

1 glass white wine

2 tbsp olive oil

1 tbsp red pesto

1 tsp paprika powder

1 tbsp lemon juice

2 cloves garlic

2 carrots

1 onion

1 knob of butter

Preparation

Preheat the oven to 180°C.

Chop the carrots, onion, and the garlic into small pieces and slice the mushrooms.

Cut the pork lengthwise – but don't cut completely through.

Season the inside of the pork with salt, pepper, paprika and rub with red pesto.

Place the slices of ham on top of the pork and layer with grated cheese.

Roll the roast tightly, press firmly and tie with twine.

Place the meat in a greased roasting tin and roast in the preheated oven for 40 minutes – regularly basting with the juices.

Meanwhile, fry the chopped onions, carrots and garlic in a pan, without browning. Add the mushrooms and sprinkle with lemon juice.

Stew the vegetables until al-dente.

Deglaze with the white wine and reduce until most of the liquid has evaporated.

Finishing

Take the dish out of the oven, remove the roasting fat and carve into thick slices.

Place the slices back into the roasting tin and pour the brown cream sauce over the stewed vegetables.

Put the complete dish back into the oven and roast at 120 °C for a final five minutes.

Slow-cooked vegetarian chilli 'sin carne' with aubergine

Ingredients

1 small aubergine

2 large onions

200g quorn mince*

1 red, 1 yellow and 1 green pepper

2 cloves garlic

3 tablespoons olive oil

250g whole grain rice

½ vegetable stock cube

1 tbsp herb mix chilli con carne

1 tin of chopped tomatoes

1/2 dl white wine

250g red kidney beans (tin)

1 tbsp chopped parsley

1 tbsp chopped chives

1 tbsp lemon juice

Preparation

Cut the aubergine into cubes, the onions into rings and the pepper into pieces.

Put the red beans into a sieve, rinse in cold running water and leave to drain.

Sweat the onion rings and the shredded garlic in heated olive oil until glazed.

Add the quorn mince and the herb mix and fry for about 5mins while stirring.

Add the aubergine and the paprika and stew until cooked on a low heat.

Pour over the white wine, bring to the boil and add the peeled tomato with the liquid.

Leave to simmer for about 20mins on a low heat.

After 10mins add the red kidney beans, stir well leave to simmer.

Meanwhile cook the rice in vegetable stock, drain in a sieve or colander and leave to drain well.

Season the chilli sin carne with finely ground
pepper, salt and some drops of lemon juice.

Chapter 6: Final Thought

Parkinson's disease casts a broad shadow over various facets of life, from professional commitments to personal relationships and leisure pursuits. Even in its nascent stages, the illness can subtly alter the fabric of daily existence, prompting concerns among those afflicted about potential dependence and escalating care needs as time progresses. Nevertheless, navigating life with Parkinson's can be manageable over the long term without significant hindrances.

However, it's prudent to ready oneself for the possibility of increasing reliance on support mechanisms. Studies suggest that individuals tend to fare better in coping with their condition when they remain socially engaged rather than retreating into isolation. Robust medical assistance is essential, alongside the active involvement of family, friends, and acquaintances, particularly when assistance with routine activities becomes necessary.

For many individuals grappling with Parkinson's, sustaining an active lifestyle for as long as feasible yields positive outcomes. Yet, in pursuing such endeavors, it becomes imperative to acknowledge personal limitations and to continuously align physical mobility and daily/work-related activities with one's capabilities.

www.ingramcontent.com/pod-product-compliance
Lightning Source LLC
Chambersburg PA
CBHW061050250726
48653CB00001B/334